FAT TO FANTASTIC

TRANSFORM YOUR BODY INTO A MASTERPIECE

By

Lynne S. Blank

Fat to Fantastic

Copyright © by Lynne S. Blank 2023. All rights reserved.

Fat to Fantastic

TABLE OF CONTENT

INTRODUCTION

WEIGHT LOSS STRUGGLE

Chapter 1

Tracking Your Weight Loss Progress

Chapter 2

The Art of Conquering Hunger and Putting an End to Emotional Overeating

Chapter 3

Is It Necessary to Diet?

Chapter 4

The Difference Between Good Food and Bad Food

Chapter 5

The Strength of Protein

Chapter 6

The Structuring of your Workout

CONCLUSION

INTRODUCTION

WEIGHT LOSS STRUGGLE

Losing weight is a common objective for many people, despite the fact that it is frequently a challenge. Changing your food, your workout routine, and your overall lifestyle are necessary steps in the process of losing weight. The path to a healthier weight can be challenging and may call for tenacity, patience, and determination on the part of the individual.

Changing your eating habits is one of the most difficult problems associated with weight loss. The consumption of unhealthy foods is a deeply embedded component of the lifestyle of a large number of people. It is essential to follow a well-balanced diet that consists of plenty of fruits, vegetables, whole grains, and lean sources of protein in order to successfully lose weight. It is essential to pay attention to the size of your portions and restrict the number of processed meals and sugary beverages that you consume.

Exercising regularly is another essential component of a successful weight loss plan. Not only will engaging in regular physical activity help you burn calories, but it will also help you grow muscle, speed up your metabolism, and improve your overall health. However, if you are not accustomed to leading an active lifestyle, it might be difficult to find the drive to go to the gym and work out. Physical activity can be made more fun and sustainable by doing things like setting objectives that are within one's reach, finding a training partner, or trying out new forms of exercise.

One of the most common challenges encountered on the path to weight loss is stress. It's very uncommon for us to seek solace in the form of comfort foods during times of high stress, which can ultimately contribute to overeating and weight gain. Finding healthy ways to manage stress, such as by engaging in physical activity, practicing meditation, or spending time with loved ones, can assist in preventing weight gain that is a direct result of stress.

Genes are yet another component that can make it challenging to shed excess pounds. Some people may have a genetic predisposition to put on extra weight, making it more difficult for them to successfully lose weight. On the other hand, this does not imply that losing weight is an impossible task. It is still feasible to attain your weight loss objectives if you are dedicated to the process and make a commitment to leading a healthy lifestyle.

Having a constructive mentality and treating yourself with compassion are also essential components of a successful weight loss journey. It is easy to feel disheartened when you have a setback, but it is essential to keep in mind that losing weight is a process and not a destination. Don't give up and remember to celebrate your victories, no matter how tiny they may be.

In conclusion, maintaining a healthy weight can be challenging, but it is not impossible. You may triumph over the obstacles and realize your weight reduction objectives if you commit to adopting a nutritious diet, participating in regular physical activity, finding effective ways to manage stress, and maintaining a good attitude. Be patient and remember that achieving your goal weight is a journey, not a destination; therefore, you should enjoy your progress along the way.

Chapter 1

Tracking Your Weight Loss Progress

The first thing you need to do is determine how many calories you should be cutting out of your diet each day.

What is Calorie Deficit?

It is a straightforward term that refers to a disparity between the number of calories that are ingested and the number of calories that are necessary to keep the body at its current weight.

To put it another way, you are consuming a lower number of calories than your body is burning. Your body is now forced to pull fuel from its fat reserves since it has no other option.

This is the only method that will deplete the fat stores in your body and cause you to lose weight.

To achieve optimal results, you should shoot for a daily deficit of about 500 calories. You don't need to be fixated on the numbers or strive for perfection in everything you do. As long as you keep your calorie intake between 400 and 600 per day, you will be healthy and continue to shed pounds in a healthy manner.

You can improve your chances of achieving your goal of losing weight by making a plan and keeping track of your progress. Losing weight is a difficult goal. If you have a thorough plan laid out, it will be easier for you to hold yourself accountable, stay motivated, and stay on the right path.

The following are some suggestions that will assist you in organizing and keeping track of your trip to lose weight.

Establish goals that can be attained: One of the most important steps in the process of losing weight is to establish goals that can be attained. This could be a goal to exercise a certain number of times per week or to lose a certain amount of weight by a certain date. Another option would be to run a certain distance every day. Put your objectives in writing and make sure you keep coming back to them so you can maintain your motivation.

Make a plan for your meals: Maintaining a healthy weight requires following a well-rounded diet. Make sure to include a variety of nutritious foods in your meal plans, such as fruits, vegetables, whole grains, and lean sources of protein. Meal planning should be done in advance. You should give some thought to arranging your meals and snacks for the coming week so that you may avoid the temptation of reaching for selections that are less healthful.

Maintain a food journal: Keeping a food journal can be a useful tool for weight loss because it helps you keep track of how much food you consume. This can be accomplished through the use of an app, a website, or a food journal. Your ability to see what you are eating, detect any unhealthy behaviors and make adjustments to your diet based on your needs are all enhanced when you keep a record of the food you consume.

Regular physical activity is vital for weight loss and should be incorporated into your exercise routine. Create an exercise schedule for yourself, and put it at the top of your to-do list. Aim to engage in some form of physical activity for at least half an hour every day, and think about trying out different things like walking, cycling, swimming, or lifting weights.

Weigh yourself on a regular basis: Monitoring your weight on a frequent basis is an effective technique to gauge how well you are doing with your fitness goals. It is recommended that you weigh yourself once a week; however, you should try to avoid measuring yourself every day due to the fact that your weight can change.

Rejoice in your accomplishments: Rejoicing in your achievements is a crucial element of keeping track of your progress as you work to lose weight. Recognize even the smallest of your accomplishments and give yourself a reward for all of the hard work you've put in. You will find that this helps you stay motivated and on track.

Monitoring your progress

Everything that can be measured can be managed. Therefore, it is essential that you track your progress and keep a tight check on both the food that you eat and the workouts that you do.

You will need to get on a scale and weigh yourself first thing in order to get started. It is recommended that you carry out this task once a week on the same day and at the same hour each week.

Do not weigh yourself every day because the results can be discouraging and your weight will likely change throughout the course of the day. It is sufficient to do so once a week, and the results will accurately represent any weight decrease.

Take into consideration that the weight you see on the scale simply provides you with a basic impression; it does not indicate your body composition in any way.

For instance, if you lost 3 pounds of fat but developed 2 pounds of muscle, the scale will only show a decrease of 1 little pound even though you have reduced weight overall. This can easily lead to misunderstandings.

You would actually have made some good progress, and you'll look different as a result because fat occupies a lot more area than muscle does.

Because of this, you should take pictures of your body once every two weeks at the absolute least. You will feel more driven after looking at images of yourself because the difference in your appearance will be more obvious to you. When compared to simply seeing a difference in numbers on a scale, many individuals find that seeing before and after images is considerably more impressive.

Get your body fat percentage measured if it is at all possible. You can ask your doctor to conduct this for you, and it is likely that he or she will use calipers to assess what percentage of your body is fat. This is an accurate figure to use as a guide, and your objective will be to reduce the percentage of body fat you have to a level that is more suitable for you.

It is also important to record the measurements of various portions of your body by using a tape measure and writing down the results. You can wrap the tape around the middle of your leg, your arm, your hips, your chest, and other parts of your body as well.

To ensure that the results are accurate in the future, it is essential that you take your measurements in the same locations. After some time has passed, you will see that the inches have decreased. Even if after two weeks of exercise the scales don't show any difference, if you measure yourself with a tape measure, it will undoubtedly reveal whether or not you have shrunk.

Muscle is substantially denser than fat and takes up significantly less volume of space in the body.
It is possible that you will feel as though you are not seeing benefits for the first three to four weeks.

It's possible that dropping a few pounds here and there will make the whole thing feel like a complete and utter waste of effort. You have a responsibility to comprehend the changes that are taking place in you. The body is changing in response. Your body's metabolic rate is picking up speed. The body is getting ready to use the fuel that it has stored in its fat reserves.

On the surface, there are no clear signs of change despite the fact that all of this is taking place internally. Because of this, the majority of women who start a program to lose weight end up giving up on it within the first month. After two weeks, the majority of people give up! They take some time off, during which they resume their unhealthy eating habits and sedentary way of life. Two months later, they make the decision to start dieting once more.

When does it ever end?

The most significant error was made here. You've just switched on the ignition, but you're already giving up before the gas pedal even makes contact with the metal. The key to getting started is having sufficient motivation. The only thing that keeps you going is your routine.

When you start your journey to lose weight, set a completion date for yourself ninety days in the future. Do not give up before you have gone without food for 90 days or until you have reached your desired weight loss.

It's possible that you'll deviate from your diet every once in a while. There will likely be periods of time in which you do not exercise. It's possible that some weeks there won't be any change in your weight at all. Continue forward despite all of these obstacles until you reach the 90-day mark.

If you despise having to start over, you should cease giving up. You are going to be grateful to yourself in three months' time. Do not give up on yourself and put an end to your hopes of losing weight before they have even had a chance to blossom. After 90 days, you should begin to observe the most noticeable weight loss. That is around three months. You have no choice but to allow yourself a three-month grace period.

Keep a weekly log of your progress and make adjustments to your food and exercise routines if it seems like things aren't getting any better.
This is the most effective strategy for losing weight without getting lost along the way.

Chapter 2

The Art of Conquering Hunger and Putting an End to Emotional Overeating

The issue that concerns modern society is that the majority of its members consume an unhealthy amount of food. When they are content, they will eat. When people are feeling down, they turn to food. They eat when they are hungry and they eat when they are not hungry... because they are afraid of becoming hungry in the future.

If you have the goal of reducing the number of calories you consume, you will undoubtedly find that you consume fewer calories than you are accustomed to. Because you are already used to consuming a predetermined amount of food on a daily basis, your body is going to signal that it is hungry from time to time.

This is to be expected. You are not close to starvation. It will take some time for your body to acclimatize to the lower calorie intake. There will be some discomfort, and it's possible that you'll be thinking about food more frequently than usual. You are going to have to show some self-control and refrain from eating. Keeping a calorie deficit at a healthy level is essential to successful weight loss.

Consider it a test that you are more than capable of passing. The management of their nutrition is seen as a significant source of discomfort by a significant number of women. The less food you consume, the less you'll desire to consume in the future. Your stomach will become smaller, and as a result, you will feel full with less quantity of food.

That might not take place for a week or two at the earliest. It could take longer, depending on how much food you've been consuming on a daily basis, but you can be sure that you'll require less food as the process continues.

Conquering Overeating Caused by Emotions

Many people who are trying to lose weight struggle, in addition to their physical hunger, with emotional hunger. It happens when we use food as a form of self-soothing to deal with unpleasant feelings such as stress, boredom, anger, or despair. Emotional hunger is a psychological urge to eat that is frequently accompanied by cravings for high-fat and high-sugar foods. In contrast to physical hunger, which is characterized by a growling stomach and hunger pangs, emotional hunger is a psychological urge to eat.

Listed below are some suggestions that can assist in preventing emotional hunger:

Determine your emotional eating triggers. If you are able to determine what causes your emotional eating, you will be better able to develop alternative coping mechanisms. Keep a log of the times and reasons you seek solace in food, and look for patterns as you read over it.

The practice of mindfulness is a method that enables you to become more aware of the mental and physical sensations that you are experiencing in the present moment. By bringing your attention to the here and now, you may train yourself to detect the signs of emotional hunger and give yourself the opportunity to respond in a more positive and beneficial manner.

Find other ways to handle stressful situations: Find healthy ways to cope with stress other than turning to food for solace, such as working out, meditating, or talking to a friend about your feelings. The release of endorphins and an improvement in mood can be facilitated by engaging in physical activity, while stress and anxiety reduction can be achieved through meditation.

Try to divert your attention away from your feelings of emotional deprivation by engaging in a different activity, such as going for a walk, watching a movie, or reading a book when you have this sensation. This may assist you in diverting your attention away from food and lessen the desire to consume it.

Get an adequate amount of sleep. Because not getting enough sleep can lead to increased emotional eating, you should aim to get between seven and eight hours of sleep every night in order to better control your feelings.

Consume foods rich in nutrients: Consuming foods rich in nutrients will help you regulate your emotions and lessen the amount of emotional eating you do. Make sure that your diet is filled with plenty of healthy foods including fruits, veggies, lean proteins, and whole grains.

Seek out assistance: Talking to a friend, a counselor, or other members of a support group can help you better control your feelings and cut down on the amount of emotional eating you do. If you want to lose weight and keep it off, having a network of people who will cheer you on and hold you accountable can be really helpful.

Ways to Put an End to Your Hunger

1. Skip breakfast.
This runs counter to everything else that you have been told up to this point. However, research has

shown that delaying your first meal until later in the day results in decreased overall food consumption throughout the rest of the day. If you absolutely have to eat breakfast, then do so, but make sure it is something that is high in protein and not too heavy. Leave the sugary cereals and the white bread out of your diet.

2. Consume a great deal of water.
It will make you feel full, which is helpful because many times individuals confuse hunger with thirst. In order to expedite fat reduction, you also need to ensure that you are getting enough water.

3. On a daily basis, consume one or two tablespoons worth of unrefined coconut oil.
It has been demonstrated to suppress one's appetite, resulting in weight loss, and make a person less likely to store fat in their bodies.

4. Ensure that you keep moving throughout the day.

When you engage in sedentary pursuits like vegetating in front of the television for hours on end, playing video games nonstop, watching movies at the theater, etc., you will invariably feel the urge to put something into your mouth to gnaw on it. Steer clear of these pursuits.

5. Consume a large quantity of vegetables.

Numerous vegetables, including broccoli, spinach, carrots, cauliflower, kale, and celery, amongst others, offer a wealth of healthful components. They are beneficial to your health and will help you feel fuller for a longer period of time, in addition to the fact that they are healthy.

6. Utilize plates of a smaller size.

This is a ploy used in psychological research. When serving less food, smaller plates give the illusion that there is more on them. Therefore, your brain will instantly believe that you are eating a lot even though this is not the case.

7. Get to bed a little bit earlier.

Nighttime binge eating is a problematic behavior that's common among a lot of folks. This is typically the case since they are awake watching TV and find that they become hungry during that time. If you notice that you are getting hungry in the middle of the night, you should try to get to bed a little bit earlier. You won't have to put up a fight against your appetites.

If you follow the advice given above, you will be able to cut down on the amount that you consume. After you have accomplished this goal, your goal of losing weight will move from being a possibility to a probability, and then it will become a reality for you. That's how vital a healthy diet is to your overall performance.

Chapter 3

Is It Necessary to Diet?

A healthy lifestyle must include a focus on striking a balance. You need to pay close attention to your nutrition and strive for a healthy, well-rounded intake of nutrients. Regardless of how healthy the other aspects of your life may be, your body will not receive the necessary support if you do not provide it with this. One of the most important aspects of keeping a healthy and well-balanced body is eating a diet that is well-rounded. Additionally, it makes it possible for you to avoid developing chronic diseases like diabetes and cardiovascular disease, and it assists in the prevention of cancer. Simply said, a balanced diet is one that supplies your body with all of the nutrients it needs to carry out its functions in an optimal manner.

The importance of nutrition is in ensuring that one consumes the appropriate number of calories on a daily basis. Because your body requires specific nutrients, you should make it a point to consume a wide variety of high-calorie foods, such as fresh fruits and vegetables, whole grains, and protein sources. You may believe that going on a diet is all about losing weight when it comes to maintaining your health, but this is not the case.

However, the food you consume has an effect not just on your capacity to concentrate, but also on how well you sleep and how much energy you have. One of the most important things you can do for your health while at work is to make sure you have a balanced breakfast every morning.

What are the advantages of being on a diet?

Consuming nutritious food is one of the most important steps toward leading a happy and healthy lifestyle. To guarantee that your body is able to perform at its very best, it is essential to consume the appropriate meals in the appropriate amounts. Vitamins and minerals are both essential to the maintenance of a robust immune system as well as the normal growth and maturation of the human body.

A good diet can help protect the human body against a variety of ailments, including noncommunicable diseases, which are among the most frequent forms of diseases. These disorders include obesity, diabetes, cardiovascular disease, certain forms of cancer, and conditions that affect the skeleton. Consuming food that is healthy is really necessary in order to keep one's body at the appropriate weight.

A balanced diet can assist in the regulation of hunger, the management of mood swings, and the promotion of physical fitness. Eating healthily presents a wonderful opportunity to broaden one's culinary horizons, as well as one's understanding of the world's myriad cuisines and culinary traditions, as well as the myriad approaches to food preparation. If you have an open mind and always plan ahead for what you're going to eat, you'll never get tired of eating healthily and you'll never have to worry about feeling deprived. Around the world, there are a lot of restaurants and food options that are good for you.

Foods That Cause Fat Loss

Incorporating foods that are high in protein, fiber, and healthy fats into your diet can help with weight management. This is accomplished by promoting feelings of fullness and boosting metabolism.

Examples include:

Leafy greens

Avocado

Berries

Seeds and nuts

Salmon and various types of fatty seafood

Eggs

Greek yogurt

Chia seeds

Beans with lentils

Almonds

Oatmeal

Coconut Oil

Olive oil

Consuming these foods will allow you to not only satisfy your appetite but also speed up the process of burning fat stored in your body.

Chapter 4

The Difference Between Good Food and Bad Food

Foods you should at no cost attempt to consume

If you want to get rid of excess fat, one of the most important things you can do for yourself is to adopt a diet that is well-rounded and nutritious. This diet should consist primarily of foods like fruits, vegetables, grains that are whole, and sources of lean protein. These meals, when combined with a healthy lifestyle that includes regular exercise, can assist support weight loss and general health.

When trying to lose weight, in addition to these nutritious foods, there are other items that should be avoided or consumed in moderation at the very least.

The following is an in-depth look at some of the meals that are considered to be the most problematic:

Processed and packaged Foods: There are a lot of processed and packaged foods that include a lot of calories, fats that aren't good for you, and added sugars. These compounds have been linked to a variety of adverse health effects, including weight gain.

Refined carbs: include foods such as white bread, spaghetti, and pastries, all of which are made from refined flour and have the potential to cause a surge in blood sugar levels. These meals typically include a low amount of fiber, which can lead to sudden increases in insulin levels and make it more difficult to maintain proper weight control.

Fried foods: Fried meals are notorious for having a high concentration of fats that aren't good for you, which can lead to weight gain and other health issues. Fried meals also have the propensity to have a high-calorie content, which can make it challenging to keep a calorie deficit when trying to lose weight.

Sugary drinks: Sodas, energy drinks, and fruit juices all have a significant amount of added sugars, which can lead to weight gain as well as type 2 diabetes and other health problems.

Meats that have been processed and red meats: They both have a significant amount of saturated fat, which has been associated with an elevated risk of coronary heart disease, cancer, and other health concerns. It is also possible for them to have high-calorie content, making it simpler to ingest more than is required.

Artificial trans fats: These harmful fats, which can be found in many processed foods, have been linked to an increased risk of heart disease as well as other health concerns. They may also contribute to an increase in body weight.

Foods that are high in sodium: Consuming an excessive amount of salt can lead to high blood pressure as well as other health problems. Additionally, it can contribute to fluid retention as well as bloating.

It is essential to keep in mind that the dietary requirements of each individual are distinct and that what fulfills the requirements of one person might not do the same for another. Alterations to one's diet and one's way of life should also be made only under the supervision of a trained medical practitioner at all times.

Consume These Vital Nutrients

The following is a list of essential items that should be incorporated into a balanced diet:

Fruits and vegetables: They include a high concentration of fiber, vitamins, minerals, and antioxidants; as a result, they are able to make you feel full while simultaneously supplying your body with important nutrients. If you want to acquire a wide range of nutrients, you should try to eat a variety of fruits and vegetables that are in different colors.

Grains: Grains like brown rice, quinoa, and bread made with whole grains are all fantastic sources of fiber, and they can also help you feel full and satisfied after eating them.

Lean protein: Foods like chicken, fish, tofu, and legumes are good sources of protein and can help you feel full and satisfied. Lean protein is a term that refers to a protein that has been stripped of its fat content.

Fats that are excellent for you: Nuts, seeds, avocados, olive oil, and other foods like these are good sources of healthy fats that can assist support weight loss and overall health.

Dairy products and dairy alternatives: Dairy products and dairy alternatives, such as milk, yogurt, and cheese, are good sources of calcium and other nutrients. Dairy alternatives include soy milk and almond milk.

Herbs and spices: Adding herbs and spices to your meals can help add flavor and enhance weight loss by reducing the need for high-calorie condiments and sauces. Incorporating herbs and spices into your meals can help add flavor and enhance weight loss.

These foods, when included in a diet, can help individuals reach and maintain a healthy weight, in addition to contributing to a wide range of other positive health effects. Instead of relying on just one item or one category of foods, it is crucial to focus on maintaining a diet that is well-rounded, nutritious, and contains a wide variety of foods.

Chapter 5

The Strength of Protein

This is one of the most effective methods that can hasten the process of losing weight.

When it comes to weight loss, the more protein you consume, the faster you'll see results. The process of digesting protein requires more energy from the body. Proteins, which take longer to digest than carbohydrates and fats, are responsible for a greater increase in caloric expenditure.

Never eat a carb when you don't also have some protein. Never eat fat without also consuming protein. Simply consuming the protein alongside these foods will prevent an insulin rise from occurring in your body.

Consuming eggs is among the most effective ways to increase the amount of protein in your diet. Eggs are widely recognized as one of the healthiest foods available worldwide. They have a poor reputation due to excessive cholesterol and a lot of other erroneous information that has been spread about them. In point of fact, it is better for you because the yolk contains the majority of the egg's nutrients.

Eggs are not only an excellent source of lean protein and omega-3 fatty acids, which are beneficial to the heart, but they also include a variety of other nutrients that are quite significant.

Eggs are another meal that many people regard to be the ideal food. Vitamin D, 7 grams of protein, vitamins B6, B12, choline, leucine, L-arginine, and folate are all found in them. Even though you may not be aware of what the majority of these vitamins are, the fact that they are what your body actually needs is the thing that really matters.

What really counts is the method by which the eggs are prepared, as well as the quantity that is consumed of them. Eggs should never be fried in saturated fat or in vegetable oil. Use coconut oil or olive oil. You can either briefly fry them or half-boil them.

Protein is an indispensable nutrient that is involved in a wide variety of actions that take place in the body. It is especially important for those who are trying to lose weight and improve their general health.

The following is an in-depth examination of the strength of protein:

1. Diets high in protein have been demonstrated to be effective for weight loss, and this benefit helps support their use. Protein is more filling than carbohydrates or fats, which means that eating protein can assist in

lowering overall calorie consumption and facilitating weight loss.

2. Protein is necessary for the development of new muscle tissue as well as the maintenance of existing muscle fibers. Muscle fibers are broken down whenever a person participates in any kind of physical exercise, whether it be resistance training or cardio. Consuming a proper quantity of protein assists in the repair and rebuilding of these fibers, which ultimately leads to an increase in both muscle growth and strength.

3. Protein is involved in the regulation of hormones, such as insulin and leptin, that play a role in hunger and satiety. This helps to ensure that adequate levels of these hormones are maintained in the body. Consuming sufficient quantities of protein can assist in the regulation of these hormones, which can lead to increased levels

of energy as well as a reduction in the desire for harmful foods.

4. Protein is an essential part of the immune system, and it plays a role in the body's ability to ward off illness and infection. Consuming adequate amounts of protein helps maintain a healthy immune system. Protein consumption at appropriate levels can assist in the maintenance of a healthy immune system and in the reduction of the likelihood of becoming unwell.

5. Protein has a higher thermal effect than carbohydrates or fats, which means that the digestion of protein causes your body to burn more calories than the digestion of carbohydrates or fats does. This causes your metabolism to speed up. This has the potential to speed up your metabolism and make it easier to lose weight.

As part of a diet that is both balanced and conducive to good nutrition, it is essential to consume an adequate amount of protein. Meats that are low in fat and saturated fat, poultry, fish, tofu, lentils, dairy products, and eggs are all excellent sources of protein. Aim to consume a portion of protein with each meal and snack in order to support your efforts to lose weight and improve your overall health.

If you don't consume eggs because you follow a vegetarian diet, there are a lot of veggies that are rich in protein that you may eat instead. You can get the same health benefits from eating those instead.
These includes:
Peas (Green)
The Whole Shebang (Edible-Podded Peas, cooked)
Corn Syrupy Sweet (Yellow)
Succotash (Corn And Limas, cooked)
Beans, Peas, and Lentils
Lima Beans (Cooked)

Fat to Fantastic

Kale

Broccoli Raab (Cime di Rapa, cooked)

Artichokes with Parsley (Globe or French)

Spinach (Cooked)

Mushrooms (White, cooked)

Greens with Collards

Mustard Greens

Broccoli

Zucchini Miniatures (Courgettes)

Garden Cress Beet Greens (Cooked)

Arugula (Rocket)

Brussels Sprouts (Cooked)

Chapter 6

The Structuring of your Workout

It is impossible to place enough emphasis on the need of adhering to an effective workout routine that not only increases your stamina but also fortifies your body and tones your muscles. Burning calories and dropping pounds are a lot easier when you do cardio. Only doing cardiac exercises is the primary focus of millions of women throughout the world. This is a mistake due to the fact that strength training is also essential for the process of weight loss.

When a person is at rest, their body will burn a greater number of calories in proportion to the amount of lean muscle mass they possess.

That very much guarantees that you'll be a fat-burning monster during the course of the day.

Your routine should ideally be structured such that you perform three sessions of cardiovascular exercise and two sessions of weight training per week.

The Benefits of Fast Cardio

When performed first thing in the morning on an empty stomach, cardio is a very efficient kind of exercise. You might have heard that performing exercise on an empty stomach is one of the best ways to speed up weight loss. The majority of people, however, do not find the thought of engaging in a tough workout so soon after awakening to be appealing.

The encouraging news is that it does not have to be an arduous endeavor at all. In point of fact, it is best to maintain things on a lighthearted level.

Going for a walk first thing in the morning at a brisk pace is one of the most effective things that you can do to lose weight. A stroll that is only 20 to 30 minutes long would be perfect.

It is expected that you would be able to carry on a conversation while you are walking. You shouldn't push yourself to the point where you're breathing so heavily that you're panting and gasping for air.

In this context, we are not striving for a high level of intensity. When you wake up in the morning, your body is in a condition of fasting because it had been asleep for so long. Because of this, your glycogen levels are low, and the food that was previously in your body is now digested.

Consequently, while you walk, your body will be compelled to make use of fat stores as a source of fuel. Consequently, your body will use the fat that it has stored as fuel while you are walking for the next twenty to thirty minutes.

This is a really effective strategy, and because it does not need much effort on your part, you may use it on a daily basis.

Your metabolic rate will also increase as a result of the morning walk, and as a result, you will burn more calories throughout the day.

You can go for a swim or ride a stationary bike if you do not want to go for a walk. Your body will burn fat as long as the cardio activity is performed at a pace that is moderate, and the results of your efforts will be worth it.

In the later part of the day, you should consider doing strength training or a brief round of high-intensity interval training. That is not a problem at all given that the purpose of the morning workout is only to accelerate the process of burning fat.

It is an additional strategy that can assist you in reaching your weight loss objectives more quickly. This approach is so simple that anyone can carry it out successfully.

If you can only muster the energy for a 10-minute stroll, then that's all you should do. With enough time, you should be able to gradually work up to 20 or 30 minutes. There is really no reason to go over the allotted thirty minutes.

If you give this approach a shot, you should notice a change in the next few weeks at the very latest.

Working out with weights

If they were to start lifting weights, many women are afraid that they may end up looking bulky and muscular like males. This presumption is not correct.

Even males have a difficult time putting on muscle. Women who lift weights will develop a leaner and more defined physique, but they will not develop a more masculine physique as a result of their training.

You do not need to be concerned about coming across as a female bodybuilder in any way.

Exercises that you perform using only your own body weight, such as squats, push-ups, lunges, dips, and pull-ups, are excellent ways to develop your muscles and joints.

It is essential to keep your muscles active so that they do not atrophy as you become older. Find some workouts that will help you tone your thighs, butt, and arms.

These are locations that frequently cause issues for a lot of different women. Strength training will give you curves and definition that will make you seem fit, healthy, and radiant, while cardio will help you shed fat and get rid of it.

A brief full-body workout that covers 10 to 15 minutes and is performed first thing in the morning can work wonders. High-Intensity Interval Training (HIIT) is the name given to this particular style of exercise. The clincher is as follows. Even if you don't move from where you are working out, you can still get a great HIIT workout.

Take, for instance, this particular example of an exercise circuit.

45 seconds is allotted for sit-ups.

Burpees – 45 seconds

Jump Squats – 45 seconds

45 seconds of push-ups are allotted.

High Knees for a duration of 45 seconds

Jumping Jacks: You have a minute and a half.

45 seconds worth of burpees

45 seconds of lunge jumps with alternating legs.

45 seconds is allotted for sit-ups.

45 seconds of push-ups are allotted.

After completing one exercise, you will get a 15-second break before moving on to the next one. You could even perform this workout at your desk if you wanted to. A workout could be completed during one of the breaks in the program. It moves at that rate. Because of the intensity of this workout, if you perform it early in the day, your body will remain in a state of burning fat throughout the rest of the day.

Your body will experience what is known as "post-exercise oxygen consumption" as a result of this. This means that your body will continue to burn calories at a faster pace for a period of 10 to even 14 hours after you have finished your workout.

It's incredible what can be accomplished in just 10 minutes.

It is best to get it done early in the day since once you go to bed, your metabolism begins to slow down significantly. You will receive the greatest possible benefit from your workout if you finish it early in the day.

It is important to note that in order to get the most out of these brief workouts, you should strive to make them full-body workouts. Perform complex exercises like squats, leaps, and pushups, among others.

Your workout will be more effective if you use as many of the muscles in your body as you can, as this will ensure that you are working out the entire body.

Don't just try to wing it with some basic exercises like curls with a dumbbell and call it a day; you won't get very far. All you have is 10 minutes. You have to ensure that it is worthwhile.

Your physique will change dramatically in just one month if you perform even three of these quick workouts every week. You should definitely give them a shot. You are going to be astounded.

Keep in mind that you need at least two days of rest per week. You have the option of breaking them up or having them back-to-back on consecutive days. It is entirely up to you to decide.

CONCLUSION

Altering your routine is necessary if you want to maintain your fitness level.

Everything that you've learned from this book should be put into practice as soon as possible.

After you have reached your target weight, you will need to maintain it by consuming the same number of calories each day. This will guarantee that you do not experience any more weight gain or loss.

To maintain your current level of fitness, you need to keep up with your workout routine.

You will always need to be one step ahead of the game. You'll need to keep going at it because a rolling stone doesn't get any moss on it.

It took you a lot of work to get to the point where you want to be with your weight loss. Make sure you don't throw it all away by going back to your old habits.

Eat well, be active, and don't forget to enjoy life.

www.ingramcontent.com/pod-product-compliance
Lightning Source LLC
Chambersburg PA
CBHW070320220526
45465CB00013B/1950